Pegan Side Dish Cookbook

50 delicious salad and soup recipes for your
lunch and dinner

Kimberly Solis

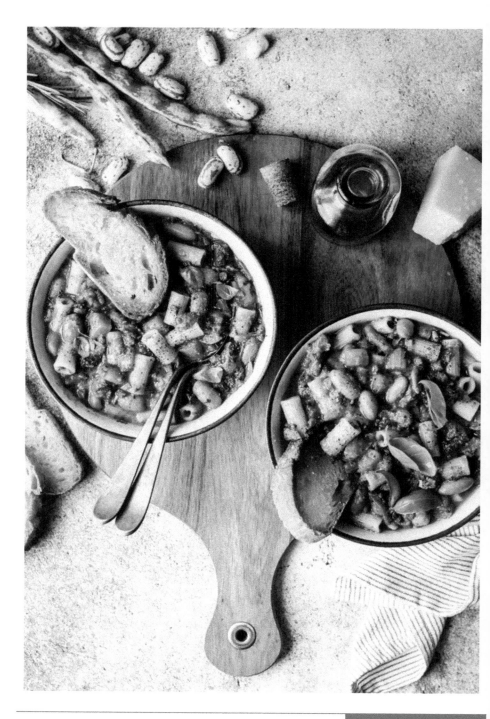

Table of Contents

BEEF SOUP 5

EASY BORSCHT 7

POTATO AND CORN CHOWDER 9

PUMPKIN SOUP.. 12

CANNELLINI PESTO SPAGHETTI 14

CLASSIC TOMATO SOUP.. 15

SCALLION AND MINT SOUP 18

KALE AND LENTILS STEW.. 19

LENTIL SOUP WITH SWISS CHARD................................ 21

SPICY FARRO SOUP 23

CANNELLINI SOUP WITH KALE....................................25

CHICKPEA NOODLE SOUP 28

GREENS AND GRAINS SOUP.. 30

VEGAN PHO 32

CREAMY SPINACH ROTINI SOUP...................................35

HOT AND SOUR TOFU SOUP 37

WINTER QUINOA SOUP...39

VEGGIE NOODLE SOUP 41

CARROT GINGER SOUP...44

CREAMY TOMATO BASIL SOUP.....................................46

CREAM OF MUSHROOM SOUP 48

POTATO LEEK SOUP 50

COZY WILD RICE SOUP 52

CURRIED SQUASH SOUP...55

ROASTED CARROT SOUP 57

ITALIAN PENNE PASTA SALAD......................................59

ARUGULA WITH FRUITS AND NUTS 61

BROCCOLI SALAD..63

BRUNOISE SALAD..65

BRUSSELS SPROUTS AND RICOTTA SALAD 67

CELERY AND RAISINS SNACK SALAD 69

DIJON CELERY SALAD..71

FRESH ENDIVE SALAD 73

FRESH SALAD WITH ORANGE DRESSING 75

GREEK SALAD SKEWERS 77

MOROCCAN LEEKS SNACK SALAD 79

MUNG BEANS SNACK SALAD... 81

RAINBOW SALAD 83

ROASTED BUTTERNUT AND CHICKPEAS SALAD 85

SALAD WITH CRANBERRIES AND APPLE 87

SIRT FRUIT SALAD 89

SPROUTS AND APPLES SNACK SALAD 91

TOMATO AND AVOCADO SALAD..93

AVOCADO-POTATO SALAD 95

AVOCADO WITH RASPBERRY VINEGAR SALAD 96

BITTER GREENS, MUNG SPROUTS, AVOCADO, AND ORANGE SALAD..............98

VEGGIE AND CHORIZO STEW 100

GREEN PEA SOUP 102

COCONUT WATERCRESS SOUP 104

Beef Soup

Preparation Time: 15 Minutes

Cooking Time: 60 Minutes

Servings: 6

Ingredients:

- 1 lb. beef, ground
- 1 lb. sausage, sliced
- 4 cups beef stock
- 30 oz. canned tomatoes, diced
- 1 green bell pepper, chopped
- 3 zucchinis, chopped
- 1 cup celery, chopped
- 1 tsp. Italian seasoning
- ½ yellow onion, chopped
- ½ teaspoon oregano, dried
- ½ teaspoon basil, dried
- ¼ teaspoon garlic powder
- Salt and black pepper to the taste

Directions:

1. Cook until it browns and drains excess fat.

2. Add tomatoes, zucchini, bell pepper, celery, onion, Italian seasoning, basil, oregano, garlic powder, salt, pepper to the taste and the stock, stir, bring to a boil, reduce heat to medium-low and simmer for 1 hour.

3. Enjoy!

Nutrition:

Calories: 370

Fat: 17g

Carbs: 35g

Protein: 25g

Fiber: 10g

Sugar: 0g

Easy Borscht

Preparation Time: 30 Minutes

Cooking Time: 45 Minutes

Servings: 8

Ingredients:

- 6 cups shredded red cabbage
- 2 large potatoes, peeled and chopped
- 1 cup peeled julienned beets
- ¼ cup chopped fresh parsley
- 2 cloves garlic, crushed
- ¼ cup red-wine vinegar
- 1 onion, chopped
- 5 teaspoons chopped fresh dill
- 2 tablespoons maple syrup (optional)
- 1 teaspoon paprika
- Freshly ground pepper, to taste
- 2 cups water
- Fresh dill, for garnish

Directions:

1. Combine all the ingredients in a large pot, except the dill.

2. Bring to a boil, cover, reduce the heat, and cook over medium heat for 45 minutes.

3. Garnish with fresh dill and serve!

Nutrition:

Calories: 127;

Fat: 0.3.g;

Protein: 3.1g;

Carbohydrates: 29.5g

Potato and Corn Chowder

Preparation Time: 20 Minutes

Cooking Time: 30 Minutes

Servings: 4

Ingredients:

- 2 tablespoons low-sodium vegetables broth
- 1 medium yellow onion, diced
- 1 stalk celery, diced
- 1 small red bell pepper, diced
- 2 teaspoons minced fresh thyme leaves (about 4 sprigs)
- ½ teaspoon smoked paprika
- ½ teaspoon no-salt-added Old Bay seasoning
- 1 jalapeño pepper, deseeded and minced
- 1 clove garlic, minced
- 1 pound (454 g) new potatoes, diced
- 3 cups fresh corn kernels (about 4 fresh cobs)
- Salt, to taste (optional)

- Ground black or white pepper, to taste

- 4 cup low-sodium vegetable broth

- 2 teaspoons white wine vinegar

- Chopped chives, for garnish

Directions:

1. Heat the vegetables broth in a large pot over medium heat. Add the onions and sauté for 4 minutes or until translucent.

2. Add the red bell pepper, celery, paprika, thyme, jalapeño, and Old Bay seasoning. Sauté for 1 minutes or until the vegetables are tender.

3. Add the garlic and sauté for another 1 minutes or until fragrant.

4. Add the corn, potatoes, vegetable broth, salt (if desired), and pepper. Stir to mix well. Bring to a boil, then reduce the heat to low and simmer for 25 minutes or until the potatoes are soft.

5. Pour half of the soup in a blender, then process until the soup is creamy and smooth. Pour the puréed soup back to the pot and add the white wine vinegar. Stir to mix well.

6. Spread the chopped chives on top and serve.

Nutrition:

Calories: 733;

Fat: 8.5g

Carbohydrates: 148.5g;

Protein: 20.4g

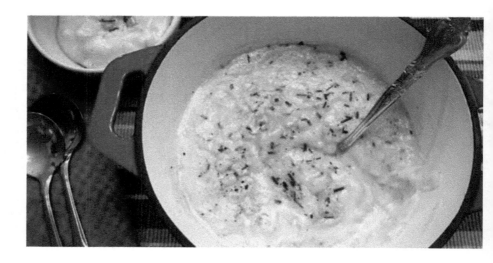

Pumpkin Soup

Preparation Time: 20 Minutes

Cooking Time: 1 Hour 10 Minutes

Servings: 8

Ingredients:

- 3 pounds of quartered seeded sugar pumpkin
- 3 cups of vegetable broth
- 2 chopped large shallots
- 3 chopped fresh sage leaves
- ¼ cup of Greek yogurt
- 6 springs of thyme
- 1 tablespoon of grated gigger
- 1/8 teaspoon of nutmeg
- 1 teaspoon of sea salt
- Pinch of ground pepper
- 1 tablespoon of butter
- 1 ½ tablespoons of olive oil

Directions:

1. Preheat your oven to 450°F. Spread some oil on a baking sheet.

2. Put pieces of pumpkin on the baking sheet. Drizzle them with olive oil, season with ground pepper and ¼ teaspoon of sea salt. Put thyme sprigs on top.

3. Roast for 1 hour, stirring halfway. Let it cool and remove the skin.

4. Put a large stockpot on medium heat, pour olive oil, and warm it. Add chopped shallots and cook for 5 minutes, stirring frequently, until tender.

5. Mix in vegetable broth, pumpkin, sage, and ginger. Season with the remaining salt and ground pepper to taste.

6. Bring the mixture to a boil, then remove from the heat.

7. Puree with a blender until smooth consistency. Pour in Greek yogurt and blend repeatedly.

8. Serve with some Greek yogurt and enjoy!

Nutrition:

Calories: 145;

Fat: 8g;

Carbohydrates: 16g;

Protein: 3.5g

Cannellini Pesto Spaghetti

Preparation Time: 5 Minutes

Cooking Time: 10 Minutes

Servings: 4

Ingredients:

- 12 ounces whole-grain spaghetti, cooked, drained, and kept warm, ½ cup cooking liquid reserved

- 1 cup pesto

- 2 cups cooked cannellini beans, drained and rinsed

Directions:

1. Put the cooked spaghetti in a large bowl and add the pesto.

2. Add the reserved cooking liquid and beans and toss well to serve.

Nutrition:

Calories: 549;

Protein: 18.3g;

Carbohydrates: 45g;

Fats: 35g

Classic Tomato Soup

Preparation Time: 10 Minutes

Cooking Time: 60 Minutes

Servings: 6

Ingredients:

- 3 pounds of halved tomatoes
- 1 cup of canned crush tomatoes
- 2–3 chopped carrots
- 2 chopped yellow onions
- 5 minced garlic cloves
- 2 ounces of basil leaves
- 2 teaspoons of thyme leaves
- 1 teaspoon of dry oregano
- ½ teaspoon of ground cumin
- ½ teaspoon of paprika
- 2 ½ cups of water
- Fresh lime juice, to taste
- Extra virgin olive oil
- Salt, to taste

- Black Pepper, to taste

Directions:

1. Preheat your oven to 450°F. Spread some oil inside a baking sheet.

2. Mix carrots with tomatoes in a large bowl. Add some oil, salt, black pepper, and toss.

3. Put the vegetable mixture on the baking sheet in a single layer. Roast for 30 minutes, then set aside for 10 minutes.

4. Transfer the roasted vegetables in a food processor or a blender, add just a little water, and blend.

5. Place a large stockpot on medium-high heat, pour 2 tablespoons of olive oil, and warm it. Add chopped onions and simmer for 3 minutes, then add minced garlic and cook until golden.

6. Pour the blended mixture into the stockpot. Add in 2 ½ cups of water, canned tomatoes, thyme, basil, and other seasonings. Bring it to a boil, reduce to low heat, and cover. Simmer for about 20 minutes.

7. Serve with a splash of lime juice and enjoy!

Nutrition:

Calories: 104;

Fats: 0.8g;

Carbohydrates: 23.4g;

Protein: 4.3g

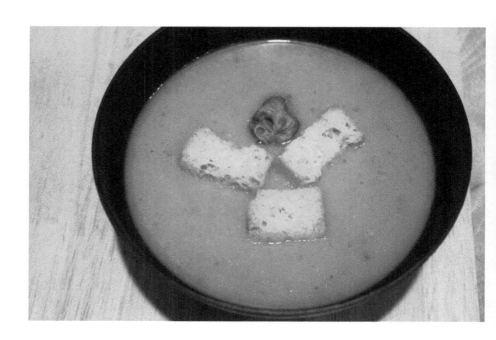

Scallion and Mint Soup

Preparation Time: 5 Minutes

Cooking Time: 15 Minutes

Servings: 4

Ingredients:

- 6 cups vegetable broth
- ¼ cup fresh mint leaves, roughly chopped
- ¼ cup chopped scallions, white and green parts
- 3 garlic cloves, minced
- 3 tablespoons freshly squeezed lime juice

Directions:

1. In a large stockpot, combine the broth, mint, scallions, garlic, and lime juice. Bring to a boil over medium-high heat.
2. Cover, reduce the heat to low, simmer for 15 minutes, and serve.

Nutrition:

Calories: 55;

Protein: 5g;

Carbohydrates: 5g;

Fat: 2g

Kale and Lentils Stew

Preparation Time: 10 Minutes

Cooking Time: 50 Minutes

Servings: 8

Ingredients:

- 6 cups (2 pounds) brown or green dry lentils
- 8 cups vegetable broth or water
- 4 cups kale, stemmed and chopped into 2-inch pieces
- 2 large carrots, diced
- 1 tablespoon smoked paprika
- 2 teaspoons onion powder
- 2 teaspoons garlic powder
- 1 teaspoon red pepper flakes
- 1 teaspoon dried oregano
- 1 teaspoon dried thyme

Directions:

1. In a large stockpot, combine the lentils, broth, kale, carrots, paprika, onion powder, garlic powder, red pepper flakes, oregano, and thyme. Bring to a boil over medium-high heat.

2. Cover, reduce the heat to medium-low, and simmer for 45 minutes, stirring every 5 to 10 minutes. Serve warm.

Nutrition:

Calories: 467;

Fat: 3g;

Carbohydrates: 78g;

Protein: 32g

Lentil Soup with Swiss Chard

Preparation Time: 10 Minutes

Cooking Time: 25 Minutes

Servings: 5

Ingredients:

- 2 tablespoons olive oil
- 1 white onion, chopped
- 1 teaspoon garlic, minced
- 2 large carrots, chopped
- 1 parsnip, chopped
- 2 stalks celery, chopped
- 2 bay leaves
- 1/2 teaspoon dried thyme
- 1/4 teaspoon ground cumin
- 6 cups roasted vegetable broth
- 1 ¼ cups brown lentils, soaked overnight and rinsed
- 2 cups Swiss chard, torn into pieces

Directions:

1. In a heavy-bottomed pot, heat the olive oil over a moderate heat. Now, sauté the vegetables along with the spices for about 3 minutes until they are just tender.

2. Add in the vegetable broth and lentils, bringing it to a boil. Immediately turn the heat to a simmer and add in the bay leaves. Let it cook for about 15 minutes or until lentils are tender.

3. Add in the Swiss chard, cover and let it simmer for 5 minutes more or until the chard wilts.

4. Serve in individual bowls and enjoy!

Nutrition:

Calories: 148;

Fat: 7.2g;

Carbohydrates: 14.6g;

Protein: 7.7g

Spicy Farro Soup

Preparation Time: 10 Minutes

Cooking Time: 30 Minutes

Servings: 4

Ingredients:

- 2 tablespoons olive oil
- 1 medium-sized leek, chopped
- 1 medium-sized turnip, sliced
- 2 Italian peppers, seeded and chopped
- 1 jalapeno pepper, minced
- 2 potatoes, peeled and diced
- 2 cups vegetable broth
- 1 cup farro, rinsed
- 1/2 teaspoon granulated garlic
- 1/2 teaspoon turmeric powder
- 1 bay laurel
- 2 cups spinach, turn into pieces

Directions:

1. In a heavy-bottomed pot, heat the olive oil over a moderate heat. Now, sauté the leek, turnip, peppers and potatoes for about 5 minutes until they are crisp-tender.

2. Add in the vegetable broth, farro, granulated garlic, turmeric and bay laurel; bring it to a boil.

3. Immediately turn the heat to a simmer. Let it cook for about 25 minutes or until farro and potatoes have softened.

4. Add in the spinach and remove the pot from the heat; let the spinach sit in the residual heat until it wilts. Bon appétit!

Nutrition:

Calories: 298;

Fat: 8.9g;

Protein: 11.7g;

Carbohydrates: 44.6g

Cannellini Soup with Kale

Preparation Time: 5 Minutes

Cooking Time: 25 Minutes

Servings: 5

Ingredients:

- 1 tablespoon olive oil
- 1/2 teaspoon ginger, minced
- 1/2 teaspoon cumin seeds
- 1 red onion, chopped
- 1 carrot, trimmed and chopped
- 1 parsnip, trimmed and chopped
- 2 garlic cloves, minced
- 6 cups vegetable broth
- 12 ounces Cannellini beans, drained
- 2 cups kale, torn into pieces
- Sea salt and ground black pepper, to taste

Directions:

1. In a heavy-bottomed pot, heat the olive over medium-high heat. Now, sauté the ginger and cumin for 1 minute or so.

2. Now, add in the onion, carrot and parsnip; continue sautéing an additional 3 minutes or until the vegetables are just tender.

3. Add in the garlic and continue to sauté for 1 minute or until aromatic.

4. Then, pour in the vegetable broth and bring to a boil. Immediately reduce the heat to a simmer and let it cook for 10 minutes.

5. Fold in the Cannellini beans and kale; continue to simmer until the kale wilts and everything is thoroughly heated. Season with salt and pepper to taste.

6. Ladle into individual bowls and serve hot. Bon appétit

Nutrition:

Calories: 188;

Fat: 4.7g

Carbohydrates: 24.5g;

Protein: 11g

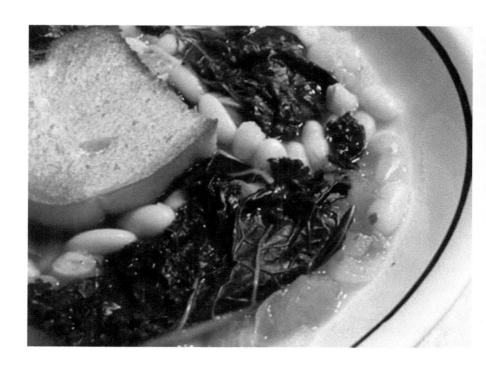

Chickpea Noodle Soup

Preparation Time: 10 Minutes

Cooking Time: 25 Minutes

Servings: 6

Ingredients:

- 6 ounces dried soba noodles
- 4 cups vegetable broth, divided
- 2 cups diced onions
- 1 cup chopped carrots
- 1 cup chopped celery
- 3 garlic cloves, finely diced
- ½ teaspoon dried parsley
- ½ teaspoon dried sage
- ½ teaspoon dried thyme
- ½ teaspoon freshly ground black or white pepper
- (15-ounce) can chickpeas, drained and rinsed
- ¼ cup chopped fresh parsley, for garnish (optional)

Directions:

1. In a large saucepan, bring 4 cups water to a boil over high heat. Add the soba noodles and cook, stirring occasionally, until just tender, 4 to 5 minutes. Drain in a colander and rinse well under cold water. Set aside.

2. In the same saucepan, heat ¼ cup of broth over medium-high heat. Add the onions, carrots, celery, garlic, parsley, sage, thyme, and pepper and sauté for 5 minutes, or until the carrots are fork-tender.

3. Add the chickpeas and remaining 3¾ cups of broth and bring to a boil. Lower the heat to low, cover, and simmer for 15 minutes.

4. Serve garnished with the parsley, if desired.

Nutrition:

Calories: 266;

Total fat: 3g;

Carbohydrates: 53g;

Protein: 12g

Greens and Grains Soup

Preparation Time: 5 Minutes

Cooking Time: 35 Minutes

Servings: 6

Ingredients:

- 2 cups sliced onions
- 1 cup diced carrots
- 1 cup diced celery
- 1 cup dry farro
- teaspoon dried basil
- 1 teaspoon dried oregano
- ½ teaspoon dried rosemary
- ½ teaspoon dried thyme
- 1 (15-ounce) can diced tomatoes
- 1 (15-ounce) can white kidney beans, drained and rinsed
- 6 ounces arugula
- tablespoons lemon juice

Directions:

1. In a large saucepan, combine the onions, carrots, and celery and dry sauté over medium-high heat, stirring occasionally, until the carrots are softened, about 5 minutes.

2. Add the farro and stir until coated. Add the basil, oregano, rosemary, thyme, and 4 cups water and bring to a boil. Lower the heat to low, cover, and simmer for 30 minutes.

3. Add the tomatoes and beans, raise the heat to medium-high, and bring back to a boil.

4. Add the arugula and lemon juice and cook, stirring, until the arugula is a deep green and lightly wilted, 1 to 2 minutes more.

5. Remove from the heat and serve.

Nutrition:

Calories: 183;

Protein: 9g;

Carbohydrates: 38g;

Fats: 1g

Vegan Pho

Preparation Time: 10 Minutes

Cooking Time: 15 Minutes

Servings: 6

Ingredients:

- 1 package of wide rice noodles, cooked
- 1 medium white onion, peeled, quartered
- 2 teaspoons minced garlic
- 1 inch of ginger, sliced into coins
- 8 cups vegetable broth
- 1 whole cloves
- 2 tablespoons soy sauce
- 1 whole star anise
- 1 cinnamon stick
- 3 cups of water

For Toppings:

- Basil as needed for topping
- Chopped green onions as needed for topping
- Ming beans as needed for topping

- Hot sauce as needed for topping

- Lime wedges for serving

Directions:

1. Take a large pot, place it over medium-high heat, add all the ingredients for soup in it, except for soy sauce and broth, and bring it to boil.

2. Then switch heat to medium-low level, simmer the soup for 30 minutes and then stir in soy sauce.

3. When done, distribute cooked noodles into bowls, top with soup, then top with toppings and serve.

Nutrition:

Calories: 31;

Fats: 0g;

Carbohydrates: 7g;

Protein: 2g

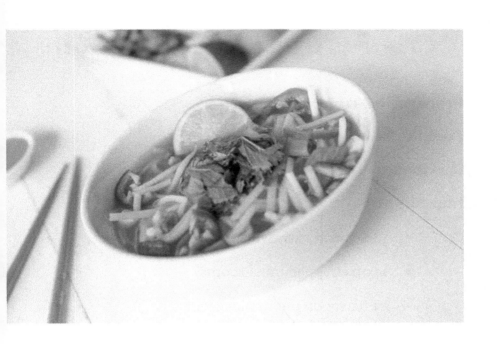

Creamy Spinach Rotini Soup

Preparation Time: 5 Minutes

Cooking Time: 15 Minutes

Servings: 4

Ingredients:

- 1 teaspoon extra-virgin olive oil
- 1 cup chopped mushrooms
- ¼ teaspoon plus a pinch salt
- 4 garlic cloves, minced, or 1 teaspoon garlic powder
- 2 peeled carrots or ½ red bell pepper, chopped
- 6 cups vegetable broth or water
- Pinch freshly ground black pepper
- 1 cup rotini or gnocchi
- ¾ cup unsweetened nondairy milk
- ¼ cup nutritional yeast
- 2 cups chopped fresh spinach
- ¼ cup pitted black olives or sun-dried tomatoes, chopped
- Herbed Croutons, for topping (optional)

Directions:

1. Heat the olive oil in a large soup pot over medium-high heat.

2. Add the mushrooms and a pinch of salt. Sauté for about 4 minutes until the mushrooms soften. Add the garlic (if using fresh) and carrots, then sauté for 1 minute. Add the vegetable broth, then add the remaining ¼ teaspoon of salt, and pepper (plus the garlic powder if using). Bring to boil and add the pasta. Cook for about 10 minutes until the pasta is cooked.

3. Finish and Serve

4. Turn off the heat and stir in the milk, nutritional yeast, spinach, and olives. Top with croutons (if using). Leftovers will keep in an airtight container for up to 1 week in the refrigerator, or up to 1 month in the freezer.

Nutrition:

Calories: 207;

Fat: 5g;

Carbohydrates: 34g;

Protein: 11g

Hot and Sour Tofu Soup

Preparation Time: 10 Minutes

Cooking Time: 15 Minutes

Servings: 3

Ingredients:

- 6 to 7 ounces firm or extra-firm tofu
- 1 teaspoon extra-virgin olive oil
- 1 cup sliced mushrooms
- 1 cup finely chopped cabbage
- 1 garlic clove, minced
- ½-inch piece fresh ginger, peeled and minced
- Salt
- 4 cups water or Vegetable Broth
- 2 tablespoons rice vinegar or apple cider vinegar
- 2 tablespoons soy sauce
- 1 teaspoon toasted sesame oil
- 1 teaspoon sugar
- Pinch red pepper flakes
- 1 scallion, white and light green parts only, chopped

Directions:

1. Press your tofu before you start: Put it between several layers of paper towels and place a heavy pan or book (with a waterproof cover or protected with plastic wrap) on top. Let it stand for 30 minutes. Discard the paper towels. Cut the tofu into ½-inch cubes.

2. In a large soup pot, heat the olive oil over medium-high heat.

3. Add the mushrooms, cabbage, garlic, ginger, and a pinch of salt. Sauté for 7 to 8 minutes until the vegetables are softened.

4. Add the water, vinegar, soy sauce, sesame oil, sugar, red pepper flakes, and tofu.

5. Bring to a boil, then turn the heat to low.

6. Finish and Serve

7. Simmer the soup for 5 to 10 minutes.

8. Serve with the scallion sprinkled on top.

Nutrition:

Calories: 161;

Protein: 13g;

Carbohydrates: 10g;

Fat: 9g

Winter Quinoa Soup

Preparation Time: 10 Minutes

Cooking Time: 25 Minutes

Servings: 4

Ingredients:

- 2 tablespoons olive oil
- 1 onion, chopped
- 2 carrots, peeled and chopped
- 1 parsnip, chopped
- 1 celery stalk, chopped
- 1 cup yellow squash, chopped
- 4 garlic cloves, pressed or minced
- 4 cups roasted vegetable broth
- 2 medium tomatoes, crushed
- 1 cup quinoa
- Sea salt and ground black pepper, to taste
- 1 bay laurel
- 2 cup Swiss chard, tough ribs removed and torn into pieces

- 2 tablespoons Italian parsley, chopped

Directions:

1. In a heavy-bottomed pot, heat the olive over medium-high heat. Now, sauté the onion, carrot, parsnip, celery and yellow squash for about 3 minutes or until the vegetables are just tender.

2. Add in the garlic and continue to sauté for 1 minute or until aromatic.

3. Then, stir in the vegetable broth, tomatoes, quinoa, salt, pepper and bay laurel; bring to a boil. Immediately reduce the heat to a simmer and let it cook for 1minutes.

4. Fold in the Swiss chard; continue to simmer until the chard wilts.

5. Ladle into individual bowls and serve garnished with the fresh parsley. Bon appétit!

Nutrition:

Calories: 328;

Fat: 11.1g;

Carbohydrates: 44g;

Protein: 13.3g

Veggie Noodle Soup

Preparation Time: 10minutes

Cooking time: 15minutes

Servings: 4

Ingredients:

- 4 celery stalks, chopped into bite-size pieces
- 4 carrots, chopped into bite-size pieces
- 2 sweet potatoes
- 1 sweet onion, chopped into bite-size pieces
- 1 cup broccoli florets
- 1 tomato, diced
- 2 garlic cloves, minced
- 1 bay leaf
- 1 teaspoon dried oregano
- 1 teaspoon dried thyme
- 1 teaspoon dried basil
- 1 to 2 teaspoons salt
- Pinch freshly ground black pepper
- 1 cup dried pasta (I prefer a small pasta shape)

- 4 cups DIY Vegetable Stock, or store-bought stock, plus more as needed

- 1 to 11/2 cups water, plus more as needed

- Chopped fresh parsley, for garnishing (optional)

- Lemon zest, for garnishing (optional)

- Crackers, for serving (optional)

Directions:

1. In your Pot, combine the celery, carrots, sweet potatoes, onion, broccoli, tomato, garlic, bay leaf, oregano, thyme, basil, salt, pepper, pasta, stock, and water, making sure all the good stuff is submerged (add more water or stock, if needed). Close the lid and cooker to High Pressure for 4 minutes (3 minutes at sea level).

2. Once the cook time is complete, release naturally the pressure for 5 minutes; quick release any remaining pressure.

3. Gently remove the lid and stir the soup. Remove and discard the bay leaf and enjoy garnished as desired!

Nutrition:

Calories: 197

Total fat: 3g

Saturated fat: 2g

Sodium: 754mg

Carbs: 43g

Fiber: 6g

Protein: 6g

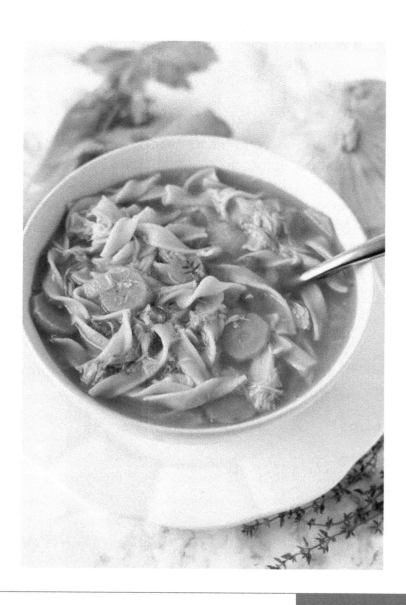

Carrot Ginger Soup

Preparation Time: 10minutes

Cooking time: 15minutes

Servings: 3

Ingredients:

- 7 carrots, chopped

- 1-inch piece fresh ginger, peeled and chopped

- 1/2 sweet onion, chopped

- 1.1/4 cups Vegetable Stock

- 1/2 teaspoon salt

- 1/2 teaspoon sweet paprika

- Freshly ground black pepper

- Cashew Sour Cream, for garnishing (optional)

- Fresh herbs, for garnishing (optional)

Directions:

1. In your Pot, combine the carrots, ginger, onion, stock, salt, and paprika. Season to taste with pepper. Shut down the lid and cook.

2. Once the cook time is processed, let the pressure release naturally for 5 minutes; quick release any remaining pressure.

3. Carefully remove the lid, blend the soup until completely smooth. Taste and season with more salt and pepper, as needed. Serve with garnishes of choice.

Nutrition:

Calories: 127

Total fat: 3g

Saturated fat: 2g

Sodium: 654mg

Carbs: 43g

Fiber: 6g

Protein: 6g

Creamy Tomato Basil SOUP

Preparation Time: 5minutes

Cooking time: 15minutes

Servings: 4

Ingredients:

- 2 tablespoons vegan butter
- 1 small sweet onion, chopped
- 2 garlic cloves, minced
- 1 large carrot, chopped
- 1 celery stalk, chopped
- 3 cups DIY Vegetable Stock, or store-bought stock
- 3 pounds tomatoes, quartered
- 1/4 cup fresh basil
- 1/4 cup nutritional yeast
- Salt
- Freshly ground black pepper
- 1 cup nondairy milk

Directions:

1. On your Pot, select Sauté Low. When the display reads "Hot," add the butter to melt. Add the onion and garlic. Sauté for 3 to 4 minutes, stirring frequently. Add the carrot and celery and cook for 1 to 2 minutes more. Continue to stir frequently so nothing sticks.

2. Stir in the stock (now is your chance to reincorporate any veggies stuck to the bottom).

3. Add the tomatoes, basil, yeast, and a pinch or two of salt. Stir one last time. Shut down the lid and cook.

4. Once the cook time is processed, let the pressure release for 5 to 10 minutes; quick release any remaining pressure.

5. Carefully remove the lid. Blend the soup to your preferred consistency. Stir in the milk. Garnish with the remaining fresh basil.

Nutrition:

Calories: 137

Total fat: 3g

Saturated fat: 2g

Sodium: 554mg

Carbs: 43g

Fiber: 7g

Protein: 8g

Cream of Mushroom Soup

Preparation Time: 10minutes

Cooking time: 30minutes

Servings: 4

Ingredients:

- 2 tablespoons vegan butter
- 1 small sweet onion, chopped
- 11/2 pounds white button mushrooms, sliced
- 2 garlic cloves, minced
- 2 teaspoons dried thyme
- 1 teaspoon sea salt
- 1.3/4 cups DIY Vegetable Stock, or store-bought stock
- 1/2 cup silken tofu
- Chopped fresh thyme, for garnishing (optional)

Directions:

1. On your Pot, select Sauté Low. When the display reads "Hot," add the butter to melt. Add the onion. Sauté for 1 to 2 minutes. Add the mushrooms, garlic, dried thyme, and salt.

2. Stir in the stock. Shut down the lid and cook.

3. While the soup cooks, place the tofu in a food processor or blender and process until smooth. Set aside.

4. Once the cook time is processed, let the pressure release naturally for 10 minutes; quick release any remaining pressure.

5. Carefully remove the lid. Using an immersion blender, blend the soup until completely creamy. Stir in the tofu, garnish as desired, and it's ready!

Nutrition:

Calories: 127

Total fat: 3g

Saturated fat: 4g

Sodium: 354mg

Carbs: 23g

Fiber: 7g

Protein: 8g

Potato Leek Soup

Preparation Time: 10minutes

Cooking time: 30minutes

Servings: 5

Ingredients:

- 3 tablespoons vegan butter
- 2 large leeks
- 2 garlic cloves, minced
- 4 cups Vegetable Stock
- 1 pound Yukon Gold potatoes, cubed
- 1 bay leaf
- 1/2 teaspoon salt
- 2/4 cup soy milk
- 1/3 cup extra-virgin olive oil
- Freshly ground white pepper

Directions:

1. On your Pot, select Sauté Low. When the display reads "Hot," add the butter and leeks. Cook until soft, stirring occasionally. Add the garlic. Cook for 30 to 45 seconds, stirring frequently, until fragrant.

2. Pour in the stock and add the potatoes, bay leaf, and salt. Stir to combine. Shut down the lid. Using the Manual function, set the cooker to High Pressure for 5 minutes (4 minutes at sea level).

3. Once the cook time is processed, let the pressure release naturally for 15 minutes; quick release any remaining pressure.

4. While waiting for the pressure to release, in a blender, combine the soy milk and olive oil. Blend until combined, about 1 minute. This is an easy dairy-free substitute for heavy cream.

5. Carefully remove the lid, remove and discard the bay leaf, and stir in the "cream." Using an immersion blender, purée the soup until smooth.

Nutrition:

Calories: 117

Total fat: 6g

Saturated fat: 5g

Sodium: 254mg

Carbs: 23g

Fiber: 7g

Protein: 7g

Cozy Wild Rice Soup

Preparation Time: 10minutes

Cooking time: 50minutes

Servings: 4

Ingredients:

- 8 tablespoons vegan butter, divided
- 5 carrots, sliced, with thicker end cut into half-moons
- 5 celery stalks, sliced
- 1 small sweet onion, diced
- 4 garlic cloves, minced
- 8 ounces baby belle mushrooms, sliced
- 2 bay leaves
- 1/2 teaspoon paprika
- 1/2 teaspoon dried thyme
- 1/2 teaspoon salt
- 4 cups Vegetable Stock, or store-bought stock
- 1 cup wild rice
- 1/2 cup all-purpose flour
- 1 cup nondairy milk

- Freshly ground black pepper

Directions:

1. On your Pot, select Sauté Low. When the display reads "Hot," add 2 tablespoons of butter to melt. Add the carrots, celery, onion, garlic, mushrooms, bay leaves, paprika, thyme, and salt.

2. Stir in the stock and wild rice. Shut down the lid and set the cooker to High Pressure for 35 minutes.

3. When there are just a few minutes of cook time remaining, in a small pan over medium-low heat on your stovetop, melt the remaining 6 tablespoons of butter. Whisk in the flour and cook for 3 to 4 minutes.

4. Once the cook time is processed, quick release the pressure.

5. Gently remove the lid, and remove and discard the bay leaves.

Nutrition:

Calories: 157

Total fat: 4g

Saturated fat: 7g

Sodium: 154mg

Carbs: 23g

Fiber: 8g

Protein: 7g

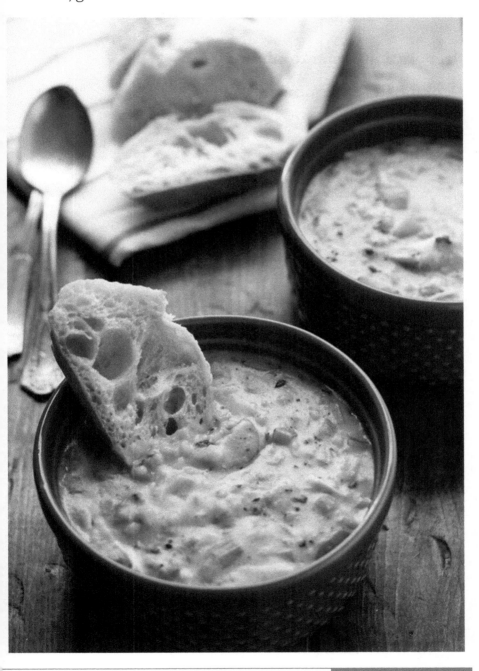

Curried Squash Soup

Preparation Time: 10minutes

Cooking time: 41minutes

Servings: 6

Ingredients:

- 1 tablespoon olive oil

- 1 onion, chopped

- 2 garlic cloves, chopped

- 1 tablespoon curry powder

- 1 (2- to 3-pound) butternut squash, peeled and cubed

- 4 cups DIY *Vegetable Stock* , or store-bought stock

- 1 teaspoon salt

- 1 (14-ounce) can lite coconut milk

Directions:

1. On your Pot, select Sauté Low. When the display reads "Hot," add the oil and heat until it shimmers. Add the onion and cook in a low heat.

2. Add the squash, stock, and salt. Shut down the lid and set the cooker to High Pressure for 30 minutes

3. Once the cook time is processed, quick release the pressure.

4. Carefully remove the lid. Using an immersion blender, blend the soup until completely smooth. Stir in the coconut milk, saving a little bit for topping when served.

Nutrition:

Calories: 127

Total fat: 5g

Saturated fat: 5g

Sodium: 124mg

Carbs: 13g

Fiber: 9g

Protein: 7g

Roasted Carrot Soup

Preparation time: 10 minutes

Cooking Time: 50 minutes

Servings: 4

Ingredients:

- 1 ½ pounds carrots
- 4 tablespoons olive oil
- 1 yellow onion, chopped
- 2 cloves garlic, minced
- 1/3 teaspoon ground cumin
- Sea salt and white pepper, to taste
- 1/2 teaspoon turmeric powder
- 4 cups vegetable stock
- 2 teaspoons lemon juice
- 2 tablespoons fresh cilantro, roughly chopped

Directions:

1. Start by preheating your oven to 400 degrees F. Place the carrots on a large parchment-lined baking sheet; toss the carrots with 2 tablespoons of the olive oil.

2. Roast the carrots for about 35 minutes or until they've softened.

3. In a heavy-bottomed pot, heat the remaining 2 tablespoons of the olive oil. Now, sauté the onion and garlic for about 3 minutes or until aromatic.

4. Add in the cumin, salt, pepper, turmeric, vegetable stock and roasted carrots. Continue to simmer for 12 minutes more.

5. Puree your soup with an immersion blender. Drizzle lemon juice over your soup and serve garnished with fresh cilantro leaves. Bon appétit!

Nutrition:

Calories: 264;

Fat: 18.6g;

Carbs: 20.1g;

Protein: 7.4g

Italian Penne Pasta Salad

Preparation time: 10 minutes

Cooking Time: 15 minutes + chilling time

Servings: 3

Ingredients:

- 9 ounces penne pasta
- 9 ounces canned Cannellini bean, drained
- 1 small onion, thinly sliced
- 1/3 cup Niçoise olives, pitted and sliced
- 2 Italian peppers, sliced
- 1 cup cherry tomatoes, halved
- 3 cups arugula
- Dressing:
- 3 tablespoons extra-virgin olive oil
- 1 teaspoon lemon zest
- 1 teaspoon garlic, minced
- 3 tablespoons balsamic vinegar
- 1 teaspoon Italian herb mix
- Sea salt and ground black pepper, to taste

Directions:

1. Cook the penne pasta according to the package Directions. Drain and rinse the pasta. Let it cool completely and then, transfer it to a salad bowl.

2. Then, add the beans, onion, olives, peppers, tomatoes and arugula to the salad bowl.

3. Mix all the dressing Ingredients until everything is well incorporated. Dress your salad and serve well-chilled. Bon appétit!

Nutrition: Calories: 614; Fat: 18.1g; Carbs: 101g; Protein: 15.4g

Arugula with Fruits and Nuts

Preparation Time: 10 Minutes

Cooking Time: 0 Minutes

Servings: 1

Ingredients:

- ½ cup arugula
- ½ peach
- ½ red onion
- ¼ cup blueberries
- 5 walnuts, chopped
- 1 tbsp. extra-virgin olive oil
- 2 tbsp. red wine vinegar
- 1 spring of fresh basil

Directions:

1. Halve the peach and remove the seed. Heat a grill pan and grill it briefly on both sides. Cut the red onion into thin half-rings. Roughly chop the pecans.

2. Heat a pan and roast the pecans in it until they are fragrant.

3. Place the arugula on a plate and spread peaches, red onions, blueberries, and roasted pecans over it.

4. Put all the ingredients for the dressing in a food processor and mix to an even dressing. Drizzle the dressing over the salad.

Nutrition:

Calories: 160

Fat: 7g

Carbohydrate: 25g

Protein: 3g

Broccoli Salad

Preparation Time: 25 Minutes

Cooking Time: 0 Minutes

Servings: 2

Ingredients:

- 1 head of broccoli
- 1/2 red onion
- 2 carrots, grated
- ¼ cup red grapes
- 2 1/2 tbsp. Coconut yogurt
- 1 tbsp. Water
- 1 tsp. mustard
- 1 pinch salt

Directions:

1. Cut the broccoli into florets and cook for 8 minutes. Cut the red onion into thin half-rings. Halve the grapes. Mix coconut yogurt, water, and mustard with a pinch of salt to make the dressing.

2. Drain the broccoli and rinse with ice-cold water to stop the cooking process.

3. Mix the broccoli with the carrot, onion, and red grapes in a bowl. Serve the dressing separately on the side.

Nutrition:

Calories: 230

Fat: 18g

Carbohydrate: 35g

Protein: 10g

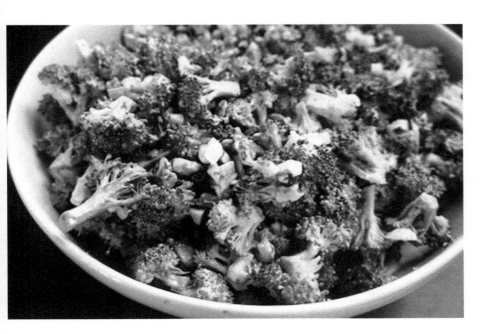

Brunoise Salad

Preparation Time: 10 Minutes

Cooking Time: 0 Minutes

Servings: 2

Ingredients:

- 1 tomato
- 1 zucchini
- ½ red bell pepper
- ½ yellow bell pepper
- ½ red onion
- 3 springs fresh parsley
- ½ lemon
- 2 tbsp. olive oil

Directions:

1. Finely dice tomatoes, zucchini, peppers, and red onions to get a brunoise. Mix all the cubes in a bowl. Chop parsley and mix in the salad. Squeeze the lemon over the salad and add the olive oil.

2. Season with salt and pepper.

Nutrition:

Calories: 84

Carbohydrate: 3g

Fat: 4g

Protein: 0g

Brussels Sprouts and Ricotta Salad

Preparation Time: 15 Minutes

Cooking Time: 0 Minutes

Servings: 2

Ingredients:

- 1 ½ cups Brussels sprouts, thinly sliced
- 1 green apple cut "à la julienne."
- ½ red onion
- 8 walnuts, chopped
- 1 tsp. extra-virgin olive oil
- 1 tbsp. lemon juice
- 1 tbsp. orange juice
- 4 oz. ricotta cheese

Directions:

1. Put the red onion in a cup and cover it with boiling water. Let it rest 10 minutes, then drain and pat with kitchen paper. Slice Brussels sprouts as thin as you can, cut the apple à la julienne (sticks).

2. Mix Brussels sprouts, onion, and apple and season them with oil, salt, pepper, lemon juice, and orange juice and spread it on a serving plate.

3. Spread small spoonful of ricotta cheese over Brussels sprouts mixture and top with chopped walnuts.

Nutrition:

Calories: 353,

Fat: 4.8g,

Carbohydrate: 28.1g,

Protein: 28.3g

Celery and Raisins Snack Salad

Preparation Time: 10 Minutes

Cooking Time: 0 Minutes

Servings: 4

Ingredients:

- ½ cup raisins
- 4 cups celery, sliced
- ¼ cup parsley, chopped
- ½ cup walnuts, chopped
- Juice of ½ lemon
- 2 tbsp. olive oil
- Salt and black pepper to taste

Directions:

1. In a salad bowl, mix celery with raisins, walnuts, parsley, lemon juice, oil, and black pepper, toss.
2. Divide into small cups and serve as a snack.

Nutrition:

Calories 120 kcal,

Fat 1g,

Carbohydrate 6g,

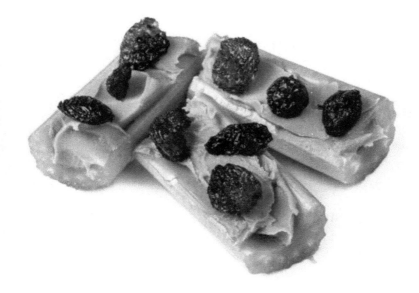

Dijon Celery Salad

Preparation Time: 10 Minutes

Cooking Time: 0 Minutes

Servings: 4

Ingredients:

- ½ cup lemon juice

- 1/3 cup Dijon mustard

- 2/3 cup olive oil

- Black pepper to taste

- 2 apples, cored, peeled, and cubed

- 1 bunch celery roughly chopped

- ¾ cup walnuts, chopped

Directions:

1. In a salad bowl, mix celery and its leaves with apple pieces and walnuts.

2. Add black pepper, lemon juice, mustard, and olive oil, whisk well, add to your salad, toss, divide into small cups and serve.

Nutrition:

Calories 125 kcal,

Fat 2g,

Carbohydrate 7g,

Protein 7g

Fresh Endive Salad

Preparation Time: 10 Minutes

Cooking Time: 0 Minutes

Servings: 1

Ingredients:

- ½ red endive
- 1 orange
- 1 tomato
- 1/2 cucumber
- 1/2 red onion

Directions:

1. Cut off the hard stem of the endive and remove the leaves. Peel the orange and cut the pulp into wedges.

2. Cut the tomatoes and cucumbers into small pieces. Cut the red onion into thin half-rings.

3. Place the endive boats on a plate; spread the orange wedges, tomato, cucumber, and red onion over the boats. Drizzle some olive oil and fresh lemon juice and serve.

Nutrition:

Calories: 112

Fat: 11g

Carbohydrate: 2g

Protein: 0g

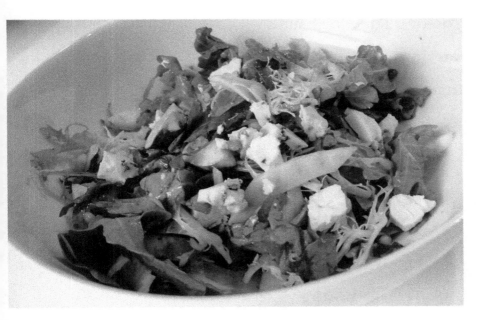

Fresh Salad with Orange Dressing

Preparation Time: 10 Minutes

Cooking Time: 0 Minutes

Servings: 2

Ingredients:

- ½ cup lettuce
- 1 yellow bell pepper
- 1 red pepper
- 4 oz. carrot, grated
- 10 almonds
- 4 tbsp. extra-virgin olive oil
- ½ cup orange juice
- 1 tbsp. apple cider vinegar

Directions:

1. Clean the peppers and cut them into long thin strips. Tear off the lettuce leaves and cut them into smaller pieces.

2. Mix the salad with the peppers and the carrots in a bowl. Roughly chop the almonds and sprinkle over the salad.

3. Mix all the ingredients for the dressing in a bowl. Pour over the salad just before serving.

Nutrition:

Calories: 150

Fat: 10g

Carbohydrate: 11g

Protein: 2g

Greek Salad Skewers

Preparation Time: 10 Minutes

Cooking Time: 0 Minutes

Servings: 2

Ingredients:

- 8 big black olives
- 8 cherry tomatoes
- 1 yellow pepper, cut into 8 squares
- ½ red onion, split into 8 wedges
- 1 cucumber, cut into 8 pieces
- 4 oz. feta, cut into 8 cubes
- 1 tbsp. extra-virgin olive oil
- Juice of 1/2 lemon
- 1 tsp. balsamic vinegar
- 1/2 tsp. garlic, crushed

Directions:

1. Put the salad ingredients on the skewers following this order: cherry tomato, yellow pepper, red onion, cucumber, feta, black olive.

2. Repeat for each skewer and put on a serving plate.

3. As a dressing, put in a bowl: olive oil, a pinch of salt and pepper, lemon juice, balsamic vinegar, and crushed garlic. Whisk well and drizzle on the skewers.

Nutrition:

Calories: 236kcal

Fat: 21g

Carbohydrate: 14g

Protein: 7g

Moroccan Leeks Snack Salad

Preparation Time: 10 Minutes

Cooking Time: 0 Minutes

Servings: 4

Ingredients:

- 1 bunch radishes, sliced
- 3 cups leeks, chopped
- 1 ½ cups olives, pitted and sliced
- A pinch of turmeric powder
- 1 cup parsley, chopped
- 2 tbsp. extra-virgin olive oil

Directions:

1. In a bowl, mix radishes with leeks, olives, and parsley.
2. Add black pepper, oil, and turmeric, toss to coat, and serve.

Nutrition:

Calories 135kcal,

Fat 1g,

Carbohydrate18g,

Protein 9g

Mung Beans Snack Salad

Preparation Time: 10 Minutes

Cooking Time: 0 Minutes

Servings: 6

Ingredients:

- 2 cups tomatoes, chopped
- 2 cups cucumber, chopped
- 2 cups mung beans, sprouted
- 2 cups clover sprouts
- 1 tbsp. cumin, ground
- 1 cup dill, chopped
- 4 tbsp. lemon juice
- 1 avocado, pitted and roughly chopped
- 1 cucumber, roughly chopped

Directions:

1. In a salad bowl, mix tomatoes with 2 cups cucumber, greens, clover, and mung sprouts.

2. In your blender, mix cumin with dill, lemon juice, 1 cup of cucumber, and avocado, blend well, add this to your salad, toss well and serve.

Nutrition:

Calories 120 kcal,

Fat 3g,

Carbohydrate 10g,

Protein 6g

Rainbow Salad

Preparation Time: 10 Minutes

Cooking Time: 0 Minutes

Servings: 1

Ingredients:

- 1 cup lettuce
- 1/2 pieces avocado
- 1 egg
- 1/4 green pepper
- 1/4 red bell pepper
- 2 tomatoes
- ½ red onion
- ½ carrot, grated
- 2 tbsp. olive oil
- tbsp. red wine vinegar

Directions:

1. Boil the egg until done (6 minutes for soft boiled, 8 minutes for hard-boiled). Cool it under running water, peel it and cut into slices.

2. Remove the seeds from the peppers and cut them into thin strips. Cut the tomatoes into small cubes. Cut the red onion into thin half-rings.

3. Cut the avocado into thin slices.

4. Place the salad on a plate and distribute all the vegetables in colorful rows.

5. Drizzle the vegetables with olive oil and red wine vinegar. Season with salt and pepper.

Nutrition:

Calories: 40kcal

Fat: 1g

Carbohydrate: 5g

Protein: 2g

Roasted Butternut and Chickpeas Salad

Preparation Time: 10 Minutes

Cooking Time: 30 Minutes

Servings: 4

Ingredients:

- 1 cup chickpeas, drained
- 1 lb. butternut squash
- 2 cups kale
- 2 tsp. oil
- ½ lemon, juiced
- 2 cloves of garlic
- green apple
- ½ tsp. honey

Directions:

1. Heat the oven to 400°F.

2. Cut the squash into medium cubes, put them in a baking tray, add drained chickpeas, garlic, 1 tbsp. oil, salt, and pepper and mix. Cook for 25 minutes.

3. Mix the kale with the dressing: salt, pepper, lemon, olive oil, and honey so that while the squash is cooking, it becomes softer and more pleasant to eat.

4. When squash and chickpeas are done, put them aside 10 minutes, and in the meantime, chop the apple and mix it with kale.

5. Add squash and chickpeas on top and serve warm.

Nutrition:

Calories: 353,

Fat: 4.8g,

Carbohydrate: 28.1g,

Protein: 28.3g

Salad with Cranberries and Apple

Preparation Time: 50 Minutes

Cooking Time: 0 Minutes

Servings: 2

Ingredients:

- ½ cup arugula

- 1/2 apple

- 2 tbsp. cranberries

- 1/2 red onion

- 1/2 red bell pepper

- 10 Walnuts

- 1 tsp. mustard yellow

- 1 tsp. honey

- 3 tbsp. extra-virgin olive oil

Directions:

1. Cut half the red onion into thin rings. Cut the bell pepper into small cubes. Cut the apple into four pieces and remove the core. Then cut into thin wedges. Drizzle some lemon juice on the apple wedges so that they do not change color.

2. Roughly chop walnuts. Mix the ingredients for the dressing in a bowl. Season with salt and pepper. Spread the lettuce on a plate and season with red pepper, red onions, apple wedges, and walnuts.

3. Sprinkle bacon and cranberries over the salad. Drizzle the dressing over the salad and serve.

Nutrition:

Calories: 70

Fat: 3g

Carbohydrate: 6g

Protein: 7g

Sirt Fruit Salad

Preparation Time: 10 Minutes

Cooking Time: 0 Minutes

Servings: 1

Ingredients:

- 1/2 cup matcha green tea
- 1 tsp. honey
- 1 orange, halved
- 1 apple, cored and roughly chopped
- 10 red seedless grapes
- 10 blueberries

Directions:

1. Stir the honey into half a cup of green tea and let it chill.

2. When chilled, add the juice of half an orange.

3. Slice the other half and put in a bowl with the chopped apple, blueberries, and grapes.

4. Cover with tea and let rest in the fridge for 30 minutes before serving.

Nutrition:

Calories: 110

Fat: 0g

Carbohydrate: 17g

Protein: 2g.

Sprouts and Apples Snack Salad

Preparation Time: 10 Minutes

Cooking Time: 0 Minutes

Servings: 4

Ingredients:

- 1 lb. Brussels sprouts, shredded
- 1 cup walnuts, chopped
- 1 apple, cored and cubed
- 1 red onion, chopped
- 3 tbsp. red vinegar
- 1 tbsp. mustard
- ½ cup olive oil
- 1 garlic clove, crushed
- Black pepper to the taste

Directions:

1. In a salad bowl, mix sprouts with apple, onion, and walnuts.

2. In another bowl, mix vinegar with mustard, oil, garlic, and pepper, whisk well, add this to your salad, toss well and serve as a snack.

Nutrition:

Calories 120 kcal,

Fat 2g,

Carbohydrate 8g,

Protein 6g

Tomato and Avocado Salad

Preparation Time: 10 Minutes

Cooking Time: 0 Minutes

Servings: 1

Ingredients:

- 1 tomato
- 4 oz. cherry tomatoes
- 1/2 red onion
- 1 ripe avocado
- 1 tsp. fresh oregano
- 1 tbsp. extra-virgin olive oil
- 1 tsp. red wine vinegar
- 1 pinch Celtic sea salt

Directions:

1. Cut the tomato into thick slices. Cut half of the cherry tomatoes into slices and the remaining in half. Cut the red onion into super-thin half rings. (if you have it, use a mandolin for this)

2. Cut the avocado into 6 parts. Spread the tomatoes on a plate, place the avocado on top.

3. Sprinkle red onion and oregano and drizzle olive oil, vinegar, and a pinch of salt on the salad.

Nutrition:

Calories: 165

Fat: 14g

Carbohydrate: 7g

Protein: 5g

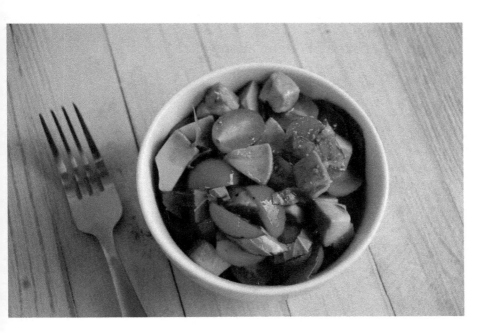

Avocado-Potato Salad

Preparation Time: 10 Minutes

Cooking Time: 0 Minutes

Servings: 2

Ingredients:

- 1 ripe avocado, mashed
- 6 Yukon gold or red potatoes
- 1/2 cup red onion, chopped
- 2 ribs of celery, chopped
- 1/2 cup sweet red bell pepper
- 1 handful parsley, chopped

Directions:

1. Steam and cook the potatoes until tender but not too soft. Stir thoroughly with all other ingredients.

2. Keep refrigerated until ready to serve.

Nutrition:

Calories: 213

Fat: 9g

Carbohydrate: 28g

Protein: 3g

Avocado with Raspberry Vinegar Salad

Preparation Time: 25 Minutes

Cooking Time: 0 Minutes

Servings: 2

Ingredients:

- 4 oz. raspberries

- 3 oz, red wine vinegar

- 1 tsp. extra-virgin olive oil

- 2 firm-ripe avocados

- 1 red endive

Directions:

1. Place half the raspberries in a bowl. Heat the vinegar in a saucepan until it starts to bubble, then pour it over the raspberries and leave too steep for 5 minutes.

2. Strain the raspberries, pressing the fruit gently to extract all the juices but not the pulp.

3. Whisk the strained raspberry vinegar together with the oils and seasonings. Set aside.

4. Carefully halve each avocado and twist out the stone.

5. Peel away the skin and cut the flesh straight into the dressing.

6. Stir gently until the avocados are entirely covered in the dressing.

7. Cover tightly and chill in the fridge for about 2 hours.

8. Meanwhile, separate the radicchio leaves, rinse and drain them, then dry them on kitchen paper. Store in the fridge in a polythene bag.

9. To serve, place a few radicchios leaves on individual plates.

10. Spoon on the avocado, stir and trim with the remaining raspberries.

Nutrition:

Calories: 163

Fat: 4g

Carbohydrate: 15g

Protein: 14g

Bitter Greens, Mung Sprouts, Avocado, and Orange Salad

Preparation Time: 5 Minutes

Cooking Time: 0 Minutes

Servings: 4

Ingredients:

- 1 cup baby spinach leaves
- 1 stir bitter greens (arugula, dandelion, watercress, etc.)
- 1 cup Mung sprouts
- 1 orange, into wedges
- 1/2 cup diced avocado
- ¼ cup walnuts, soaked
- 2 tbsp. extra-virgin olive oil
- 1 tbsp. lemon juice
- 1 tsp. lemon zest
- Fresh cracked black pepper to taste
- 1 Tbsp. tahini
- 1/2 tsp. diced fresh ginger

Directions:

1. Mix spinach leaves, bitter greens, and Mung sprouts in a bowl. Add the orange and avocado. In another bowl, whisk the lemon juice, olive oil, lemon zest, salt, pepper, ginger, and tahini.

2. Pour the dressing over the salad and toss to coat. Trim with the chopped walnuts and serve immediately.

Nutrition:

Calories: 173

Fat: 4g

Carbohydrate: 15g

Protein: 9g

Veggie and Chorizo Stew

Preparation Time: 10 Minutes

Cooking Time: 30 Minutes

Servings: 4

Ingredients:

- 1 yellow onion, chopped
- 1 tbsp. coconut oil
- 2 chorizo sausages, skinless and thinly sliced
- 1 red bell pepper, chopped
- 1 carrot, thinly sliced
- 2 white potatoes, chopped
- 1 celery stick, chopped
- 1 tomato, chopped
- 2 garlic cloves, finely minced
- 2 cups chicken broth
- 1 tbsp. lemon juice
- Salt and black pepper to taste
- 1 zucchini, cut
- A handful parsley leaves, finely chopped

Directions:

1. Heat up a pan with the oil over medium-high heat, add chorizo, onion, celery and carrot, stir and cook for 3 minutes.

2. Add red bell pepper, tomatoes, garlic, and potato, stir and cook 1 minute.

3. Add lemon juice, stock, salt, and pepper, stir, bring to a boil, cover pan, reduce heat to medium and cook for 10 minutes.

4. Add zucchini, stir, cover again and cook for ten more minutes.

5. Uncover pan, cook the stew for 2 minutes more stirring often.

6. Add parsley, stir, take off heat, transfer to dishes and serve.

7. Enjoy!

Nutrition:

Calories: 420

Fat: 12g

Carbs: 45g

Protein: 33.2g

Fiber: 11g

Sugar: 0g

Green Pea Soup

Preparation Time: 5 Minutes

Cooking Time: 50 Minutes

Servings: 6

Ingredients:

- 1 (16-ounce) package dried green split peas, soaked overnight
- 5 cups vegetable broth or water
- 2 teaspoons garlic powder
- 2 teaspoons onion powder
- 1 teaspoon dried oregano
- 1 teaspoon dried thyme
- ¼ teaspoon freshly ground black pepper

Directions:

1. In a large stockpot, combine the split peas, broth, garlic powder, onion powder, oregano, thyme, and pepper. Bring to a boil over medium-high heat.

2. Cover, reduce the heat to medium-low, and simmer for 45 minutes, stirring every 5 to 10 minutes. Serve warm.

Nutrition:

Calories: 297;

Fat: 2g;

Carbohydrates: 48g;

Protein: 23g

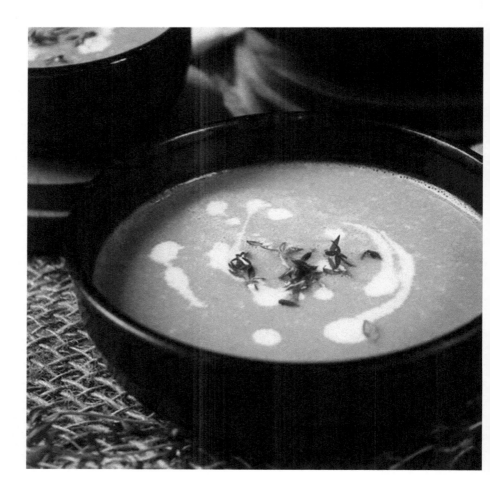

Coconut Watercress Soup

Preparation Time: 10 Minutes

Cooking Time: 20 Minutes

Servings: 4

Ingredients:

- 1 teaspoon coconut oil

- 1 onion, diced

- 2 cups fresh or frozen peas

- 6 cups water, or vegetable stock

- 1 cup fresh watercress, chopped

- 1 tablespoon fresh mint, chopped

- Pinch sea salt

- Pinch freshly ground black pepper

- ¾ cup coconut milk

Directions:

1. Preparing the Ingredients.

2. Melt the coconut oil in a large pot over medium-high heat. Add the onion and cook until soft for about 5 minutes, then add the peas and water. Bring to a boil, lower the heat, then add the watercress, mint, salt, and pepper.

3. Cover and simmer for 5 minutes. Stir in the coconut milk.

4. Finish and serve

5. Purée the soup until smooth in a blender or with an immersion blender.

6. Try this soup with any other fresh, leafy green— anything from spinach to collard greens to arugula to Swiss chard.

Nutrition:

Calories: 178;

Fat: 10g;

Protein: 6g;

Carbohydrates: 18g

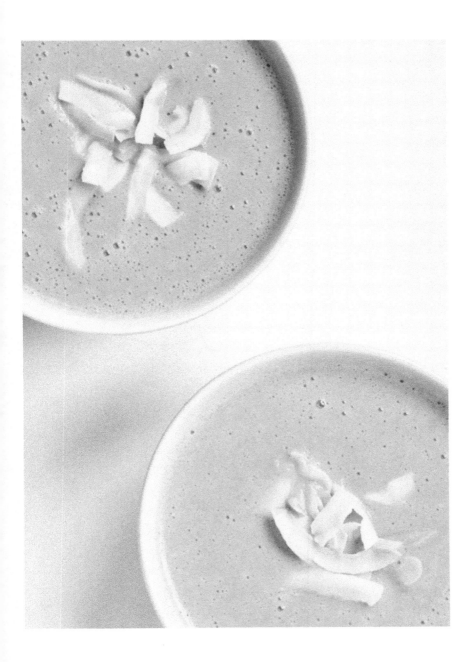